yogamo s

teaching to the mind, body and spirit

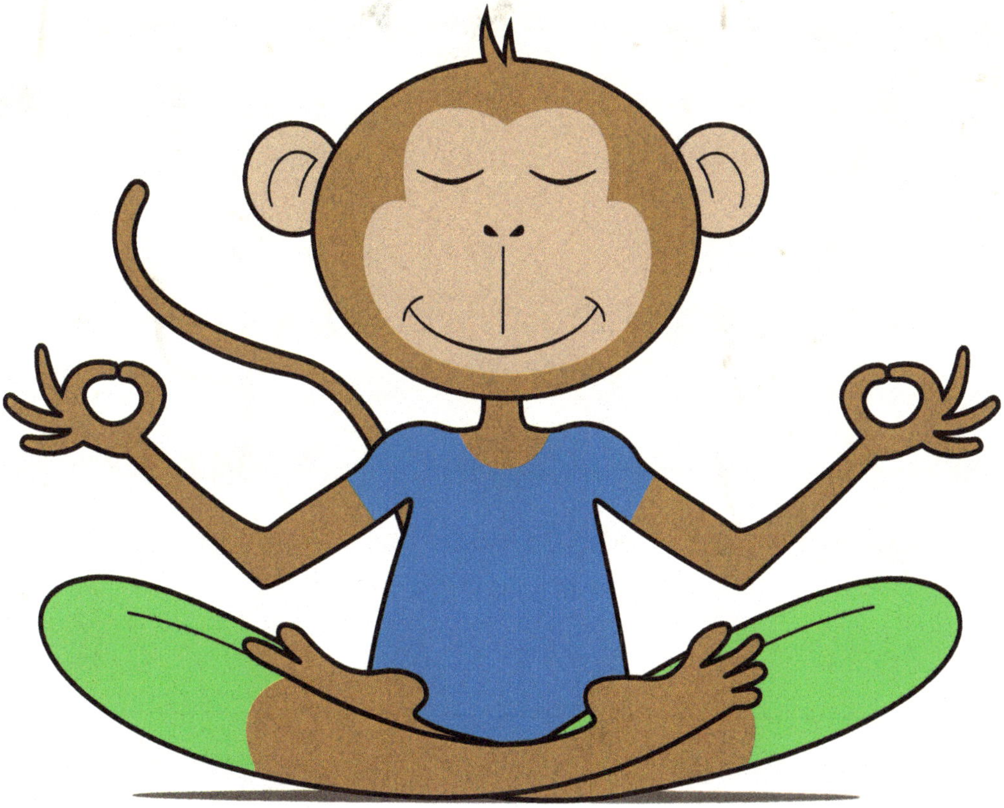

To Carlo —
My favorite doc!
And the only
neurologist with a
great sense of humor!
Thank you for
all your care.
Love,
Candace

By Candace Stromberg
Illustrations by Stewart Andrews

Page Publishing • New York

PAGE PUBLISHING, INC.
New York, NY

First originally published by Page Publishing, Inc. 2016

ISBN 978-1-68348-752-4 (Paperback)
ISBN 978-1-68348-753-1 (Digital)

Printed in the United States of America

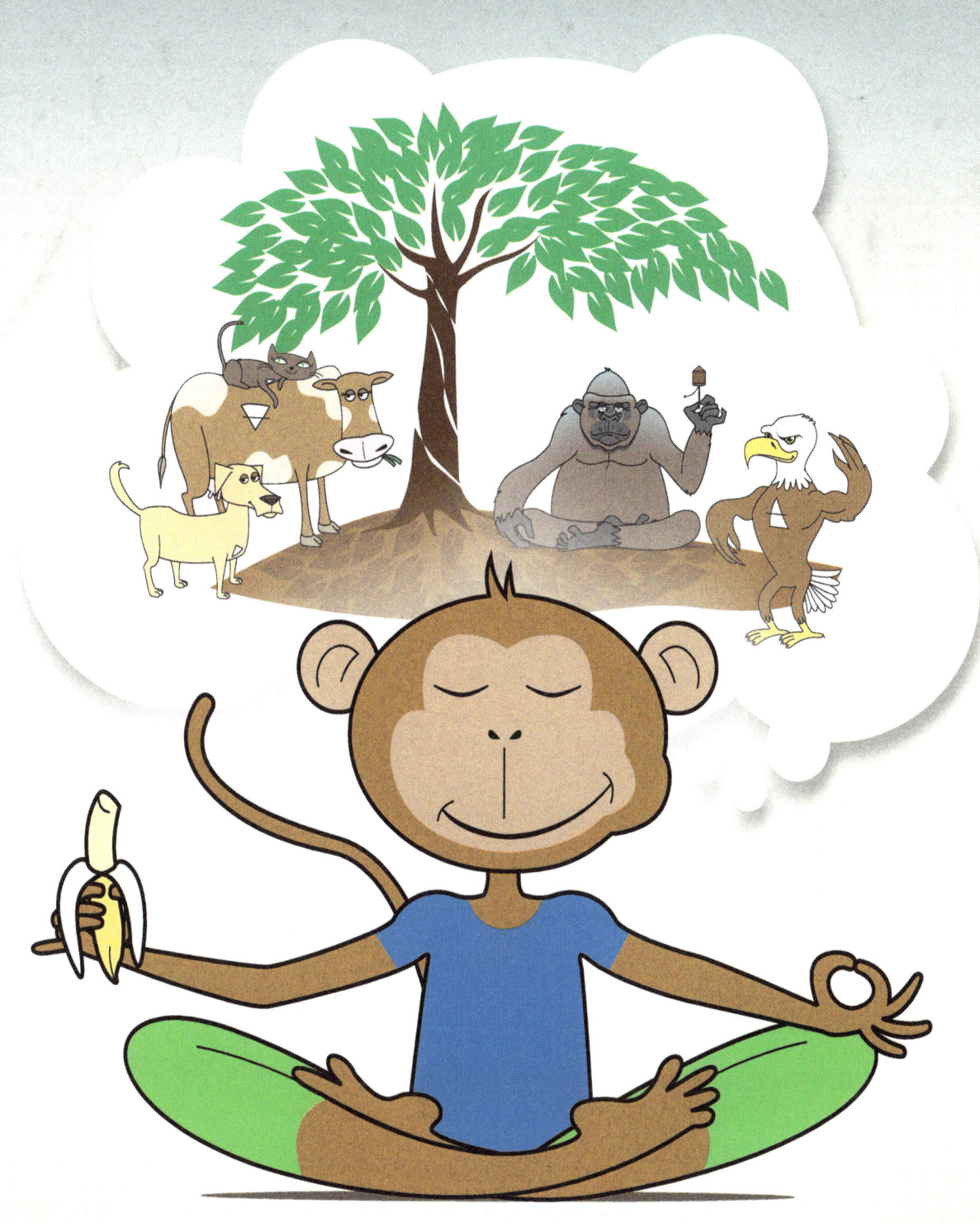

Hi! I'm Yokey the Yoga Monkey.
I love doing yoga and sharing all
I've learned with family and friends.

1

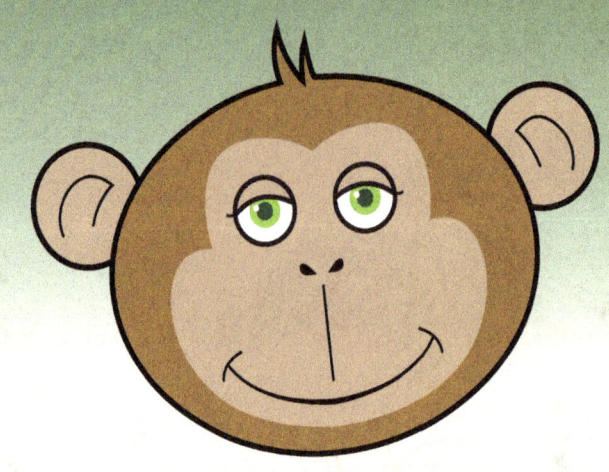

Before we get started you will need a few things for a safe yoga experience.

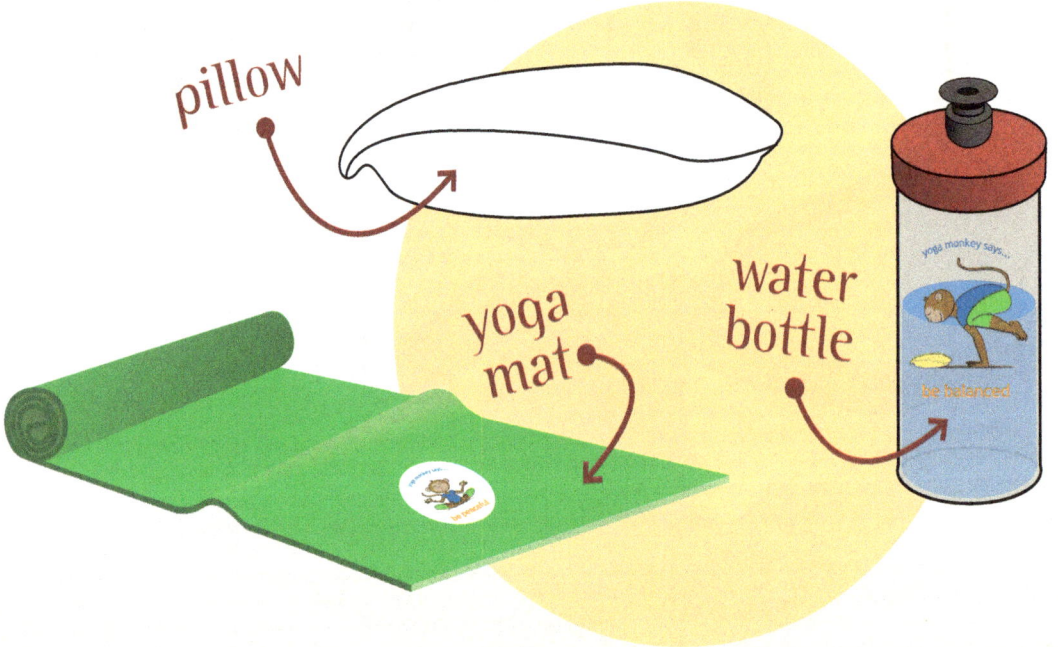

pillow

yoga mat

water bottle

Let's go learn about yoga and what it means to practice this happy and healthy exercise.

2

What is Yoga?

Yoga means "union," and "to join."

Yoga is a mind, body and spirit connection. When you join all three together, you will have harmony, peace and joy.

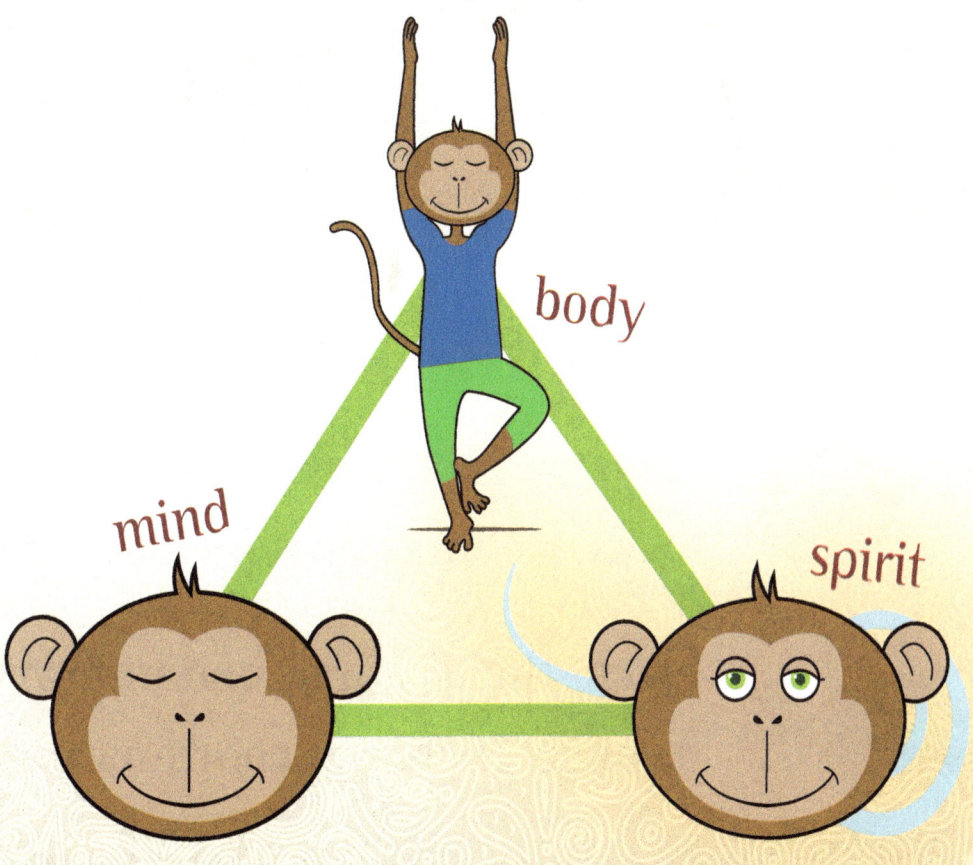

body

mind

spirit

3

Yoga Poses

Early *Yogis* were people who watched and imitated animals and nature in order to stay strong and be healthy.

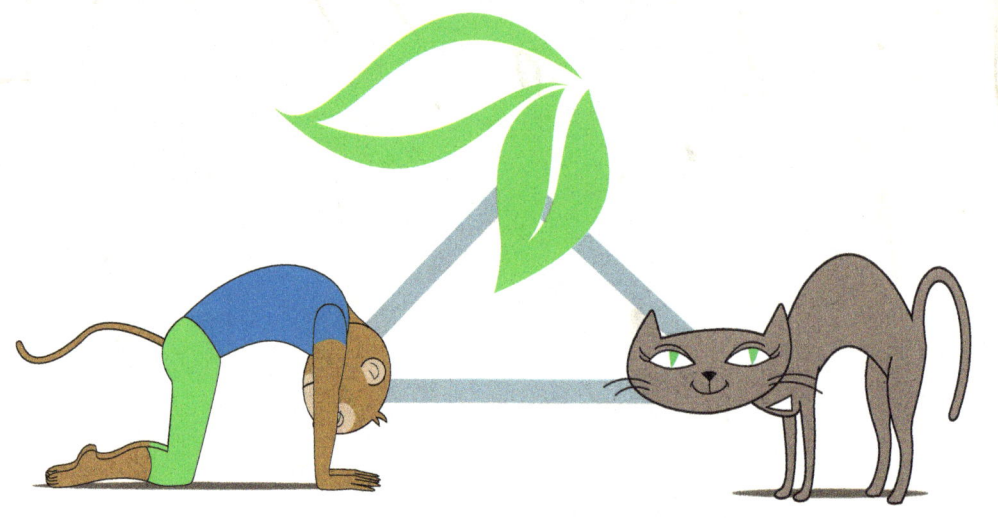

Benefits of Yoga

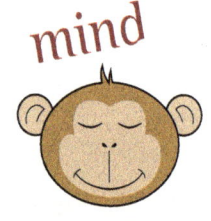

mind

Improves concentration and focus. Relieves tension and stress.

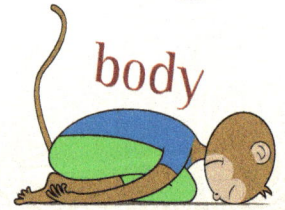

body

Strengthens, aligns and improves balance. Increases coordination.

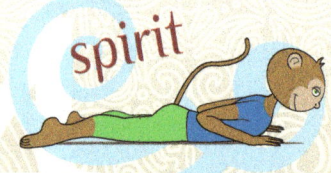

spirit

Connection to nature and self. Creates feelings of joy.

Why Yoga Is Awesome

- ☼ You can do it anywhere, anytime!

- ☼ Yoga promotes a lifetime of health and wellness.

- ☼ It helps you to develop a strong and flexible body.

- ☼ Yoga reduces injury and increases performance in other sports you play.

- ☼ Yoga boosts your immune system, a fancy way to say it helps to keep colds away!

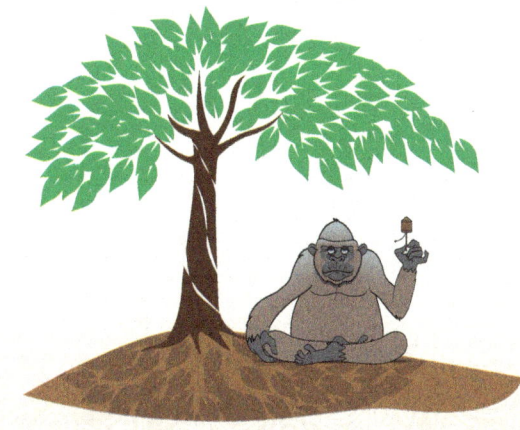

- ☼ It helps you to manage stress.

"Your mind, body and spirit are one. Treat them with love and kindness.

Papa Gorilla

- ☼ It is an exercise that is fun to do!

5

Set An Affirmation for Your Practice

You've heard the saying "you are what you eat" but did you know that *"you are what you think"?*

Affirmations [af-er-**mey**-sh*uh* ns] are positive thoughts you say to yourself or out loud. These messages are self-empowering and assist in pushing us towards our goals.

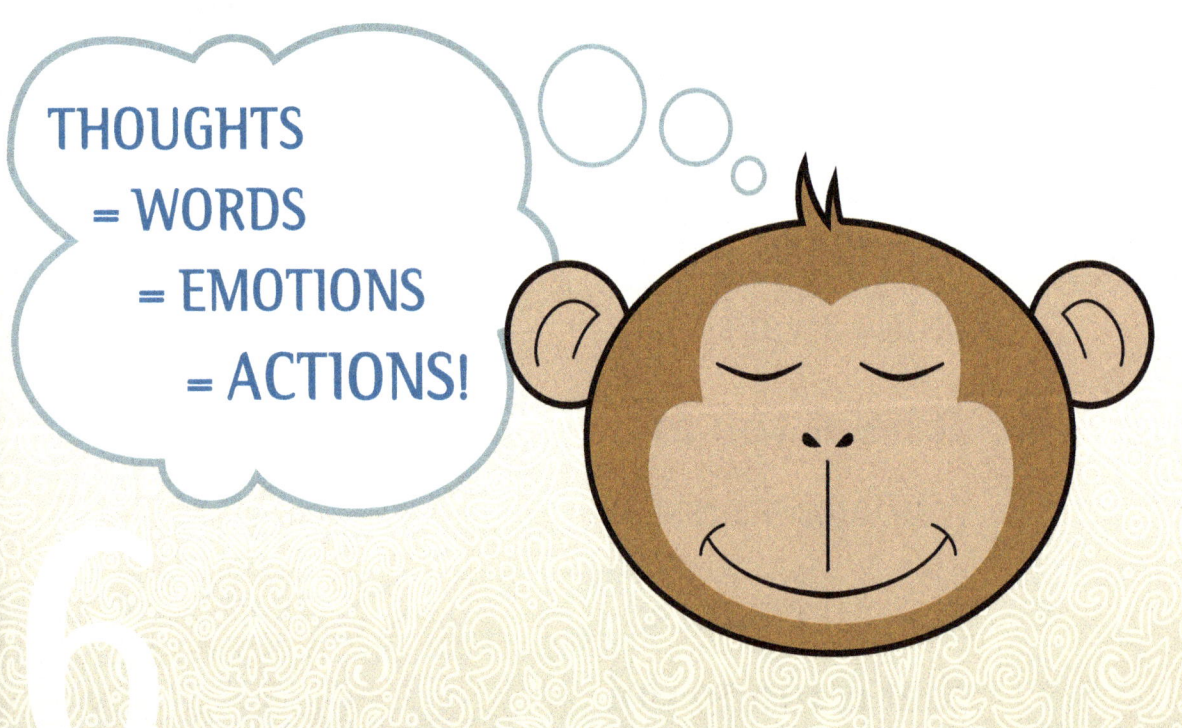

THOUGHTS
= WORDS
= EMOTIONS
= ACTIONS!

6

Emotion	Try These Poses	Affirmation
Happy	Downward Dog Butterfly	I am free to love. Laughter is good for my spirit.
Energetic/ Focused	Downward Dog Plank Butterfly	I am full of life! Energy equals strength.
Shy	Warrior Tree Plank	I am confident. I enjoy new people, places and things. I am courageous and stand up for myself.
Sad	Butterfly Child's Pose	I open my heart. I bring in joy. I create my own happiness.
Scared/ afraid	Warrior Mountain	I am strong. I am brave. I am in control.
Frustrated	Easy Pose Child's Pose Tree	I am in control. When I pause, I can concentrate and breathe.
Bored	Forward Bend Cat and Cow	Creative energy guides me to new places. Learning is fun! Challenges are healthy.

Know Your

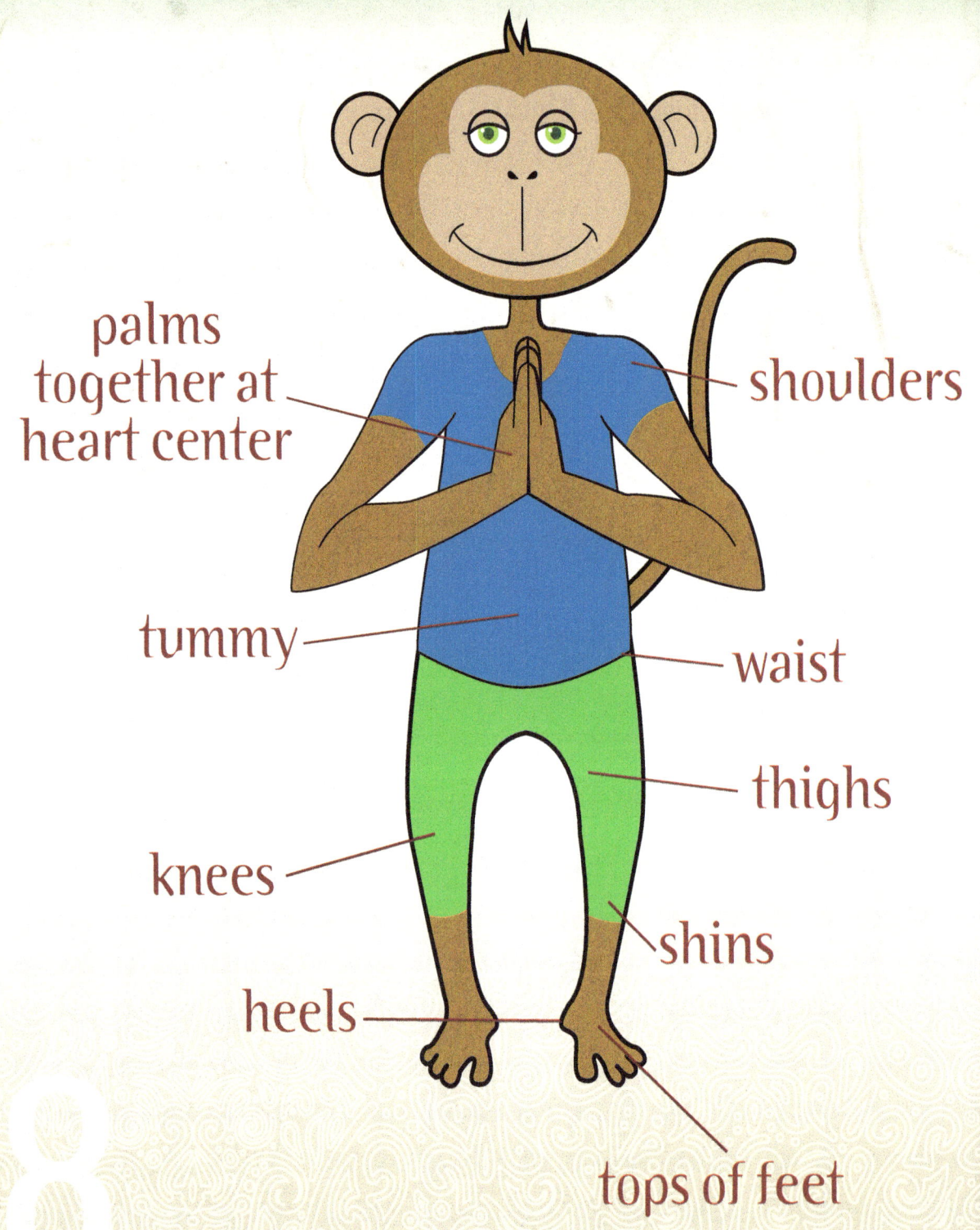

palms together at heart center

shoulders

tummy

waist

thighs

knees

shins

heels

tops of feet

8

Body Parts

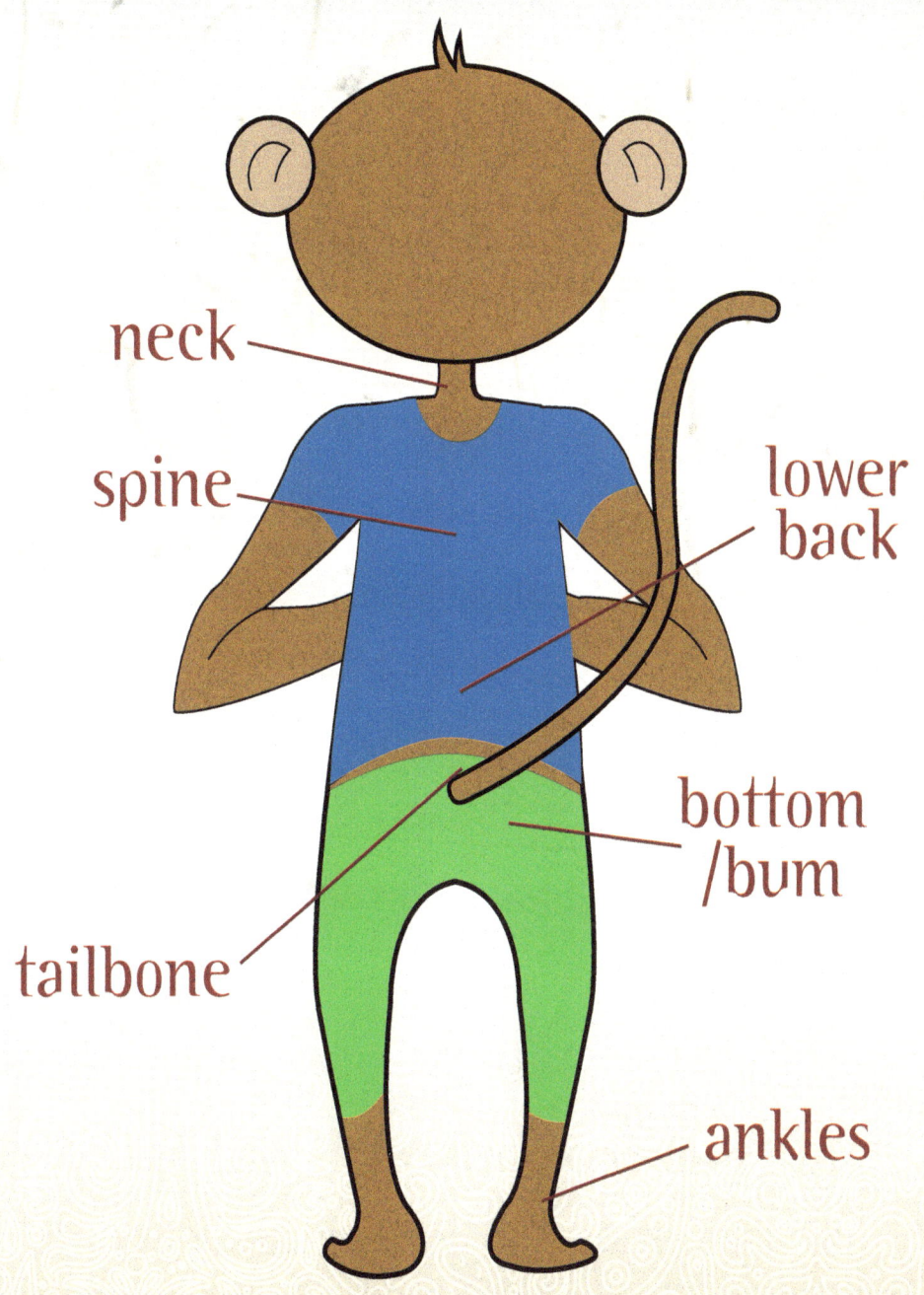

neck

spine

lower back

tailbone

bottom /bum

ankles

9

How to Use This Book

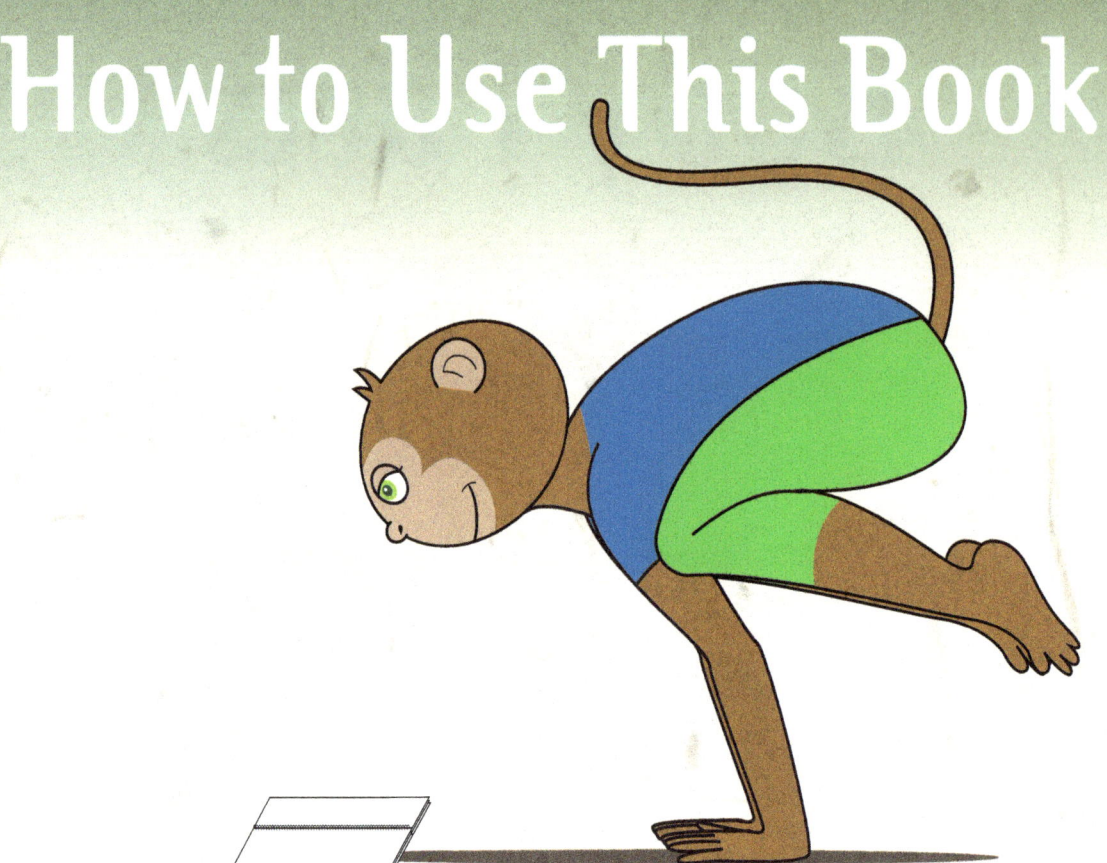

This book is designed to teach and guide you through each pose. Read and practice each pose before moving to the next page. Have a parent or adult help you the first few times.

Once you feel comfortable with the poses you may do them in any sequence you like to create your own flow.

Pose In Focus

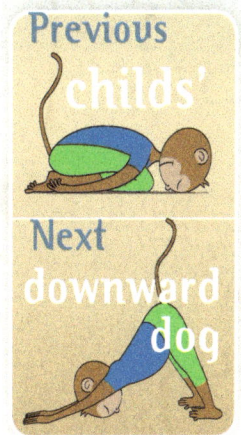
Previous
childs'
Next
downward
dog

Previous/Next

Previous and next poses are located on each page to help guide you.

Try-Its

Variations on how to do the pose or alter the pose. Kick it up a monkey-notch, you can do it!

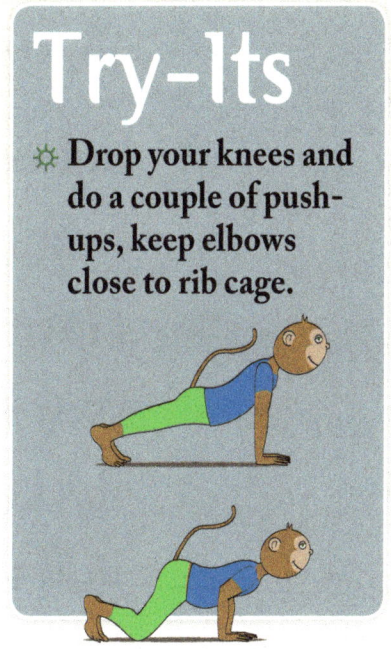
Try-Its

☼ Drop your knees and do a couple of push-ups, keep elbows close to rib cage.

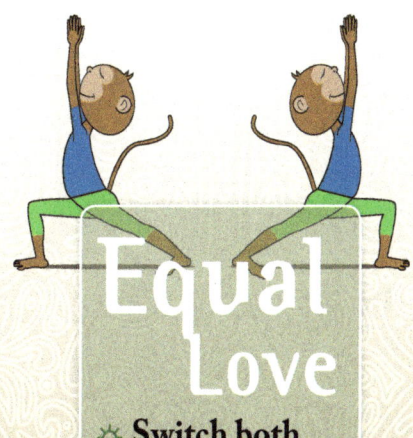
Equal Love

☼ Switch both arms and legs

Equal Love

Make sure to do the pose on both sides of your body.

11

12 Mountain ▲

Strong, Tall, Majestic

- ☀ Stand tall with feet slightly apart and heels turned out.

- ☀ Squeeze thighs and feel your knees lift.

- ☀ Have a slight bend to your knees.

- ☀ Relax your shoulders.

- ☀ Pull your belly in and up.

- ☀ Breathe slowly in through your nose and out through your mouth.

- ☀ Be as still and strong as a mountain!

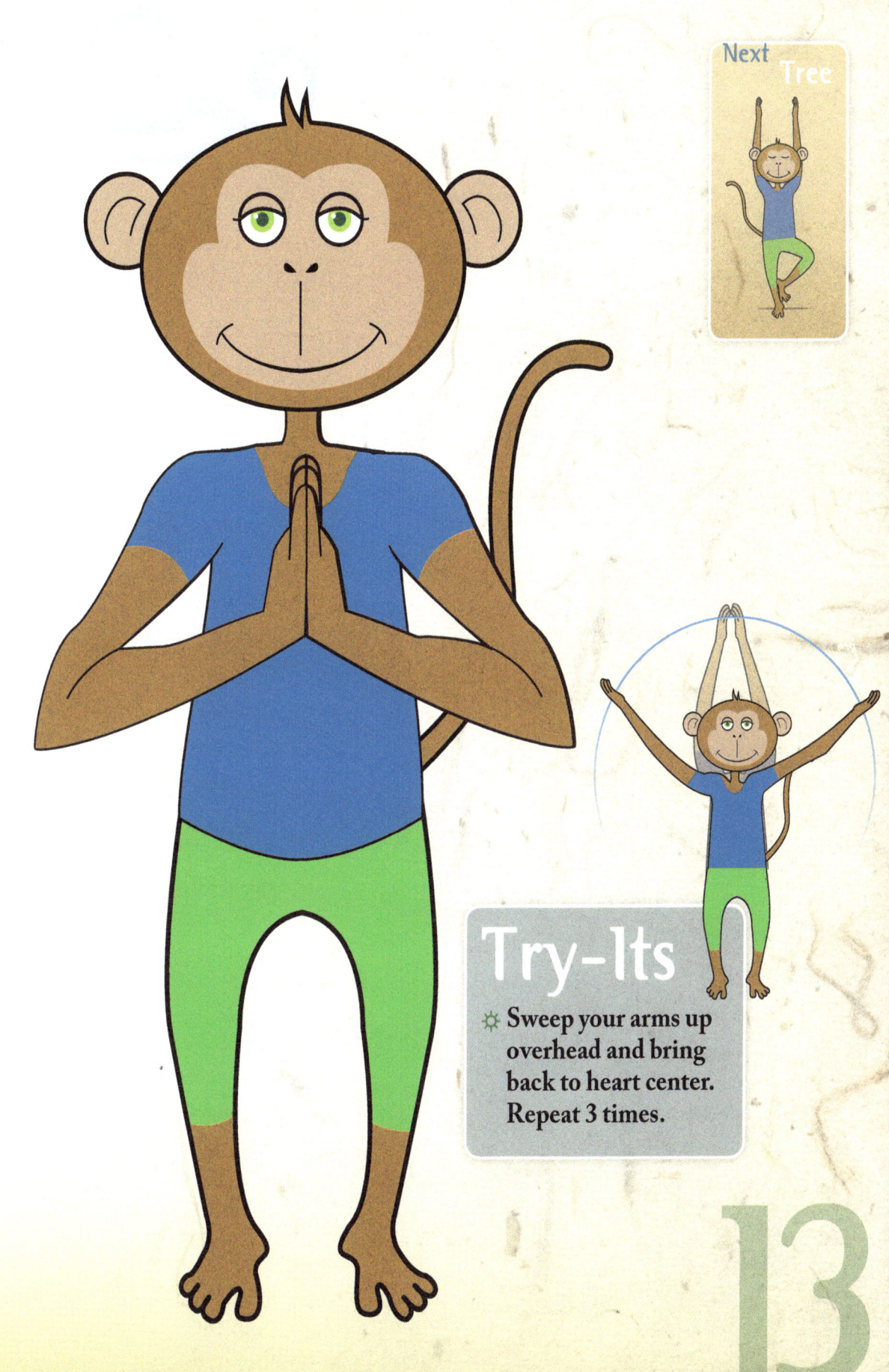

Next
Tree

Try-Its

☼ Sweep your arms up
overhead and bring
back to heart center.
Repeat 3 times.

13

Tree

*Sturdy, Rooted in Earth,
Growing towards the Sun*

- ☼ Stand tall and balance on one foot.

- ☼ To help balance, imagine roots growing down your legs, out the bottoms of your feet and into the earth.

- ☼ Place your other foot at your ankle, shin or upper thigh, do not place on your knee!

- ☼ Make sure the bent knee is facing out and not in front of you.

- ☼ Use your arms for balance — off to sides or above your head.

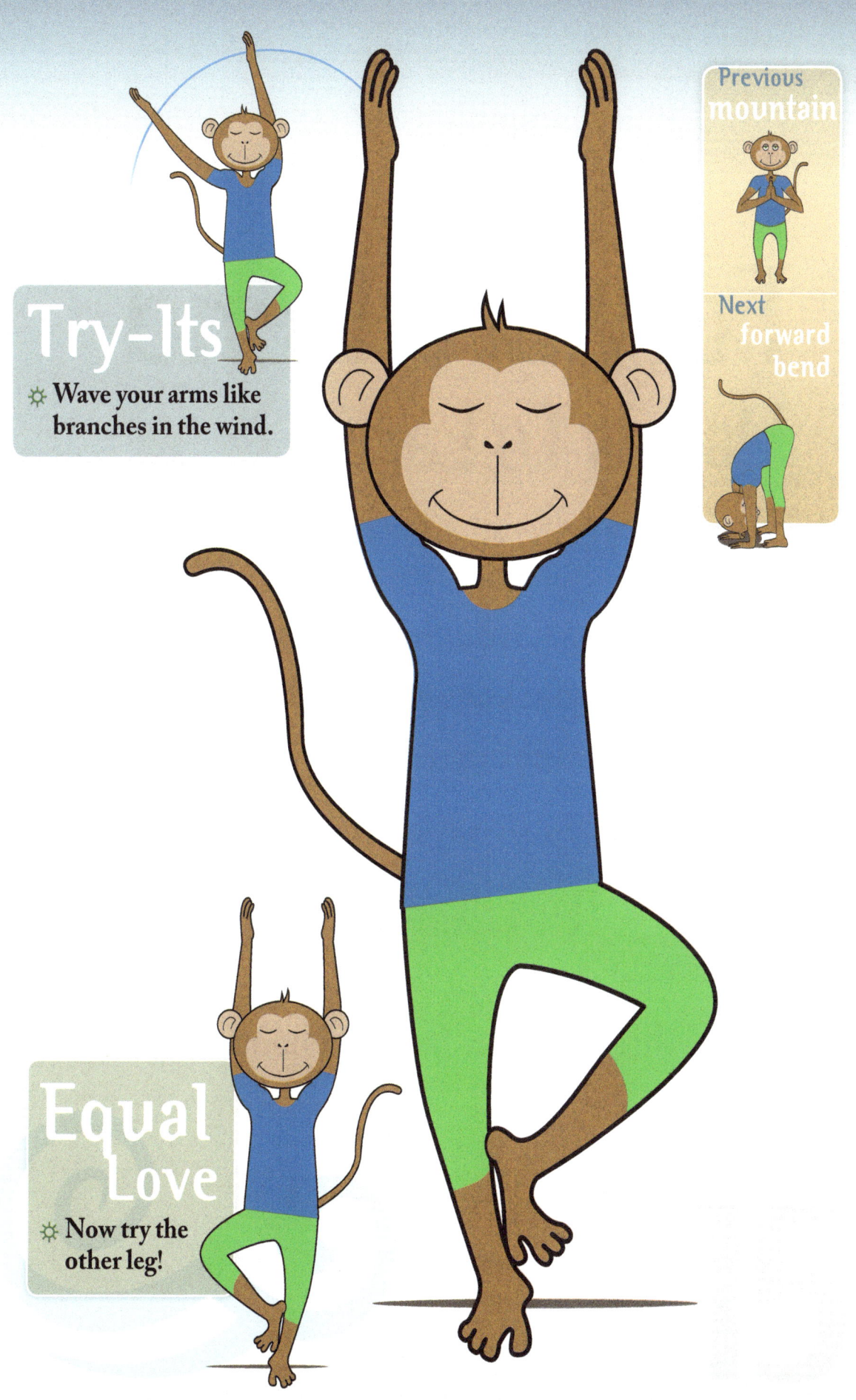

Try-Its
☀ **Wave your arms like branches in the wind.**

Previous
mountain

Next
forward bend

Equal Love
☀ **Now try the other leg!**

16
Forward Bend
Hands To Earth 🖐🖐

- ☼ Feet apart and bend at waist. See if you can get your hands flat on the earth.

- ☼ Keep knees slightly bent.

- ☼ Relax your shoulders.

- ☼ Feel the connection to the earth through your feet and hands.

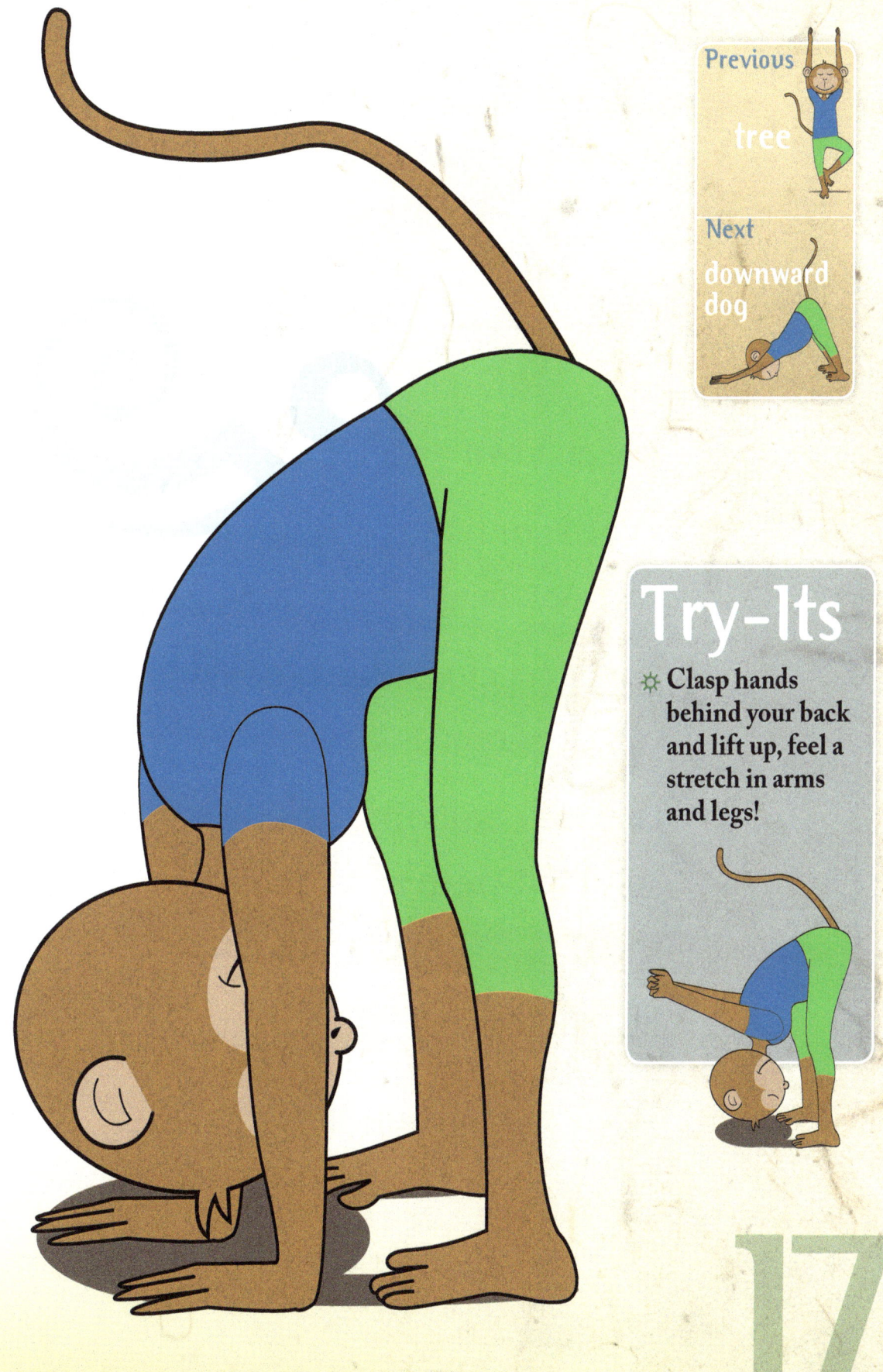

Previous

tree

Next

downward dog

Try-Its

☀ Clasp hands behind your back and lift up, feel a stretch in arms and legs!

17

Downward Dog

Playful and Happy

- ☼ Kneel down on all fours.

- ☼ Slide your hands way out in front and look back at your toes.

- ☼ Keep feet close, don't spread your legs out.

- ☼ Lift your tailbone to the sky so your body is in a "V" shape.

- ☼ Keep arms and legs straight.

- ☼ Push your heels towards the earth.

- ☼ Wag your tail and "Bark!"

Try-Its

☼ **Lift one leg at a time as high as you can go!**

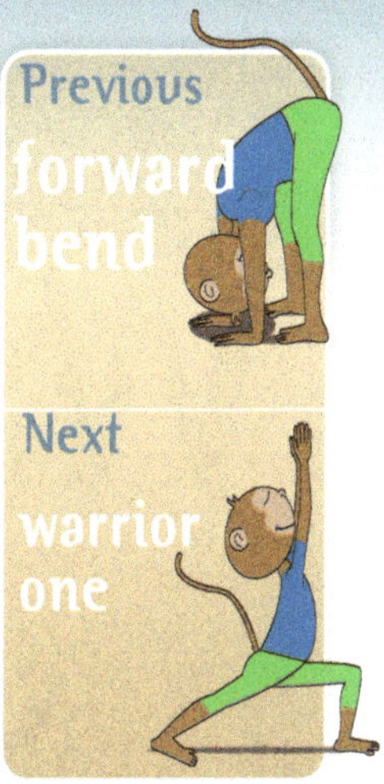

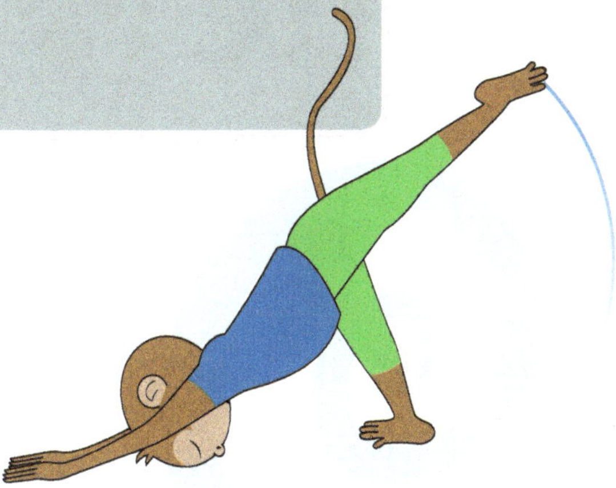

Previous

forward bend

Next

warrior one

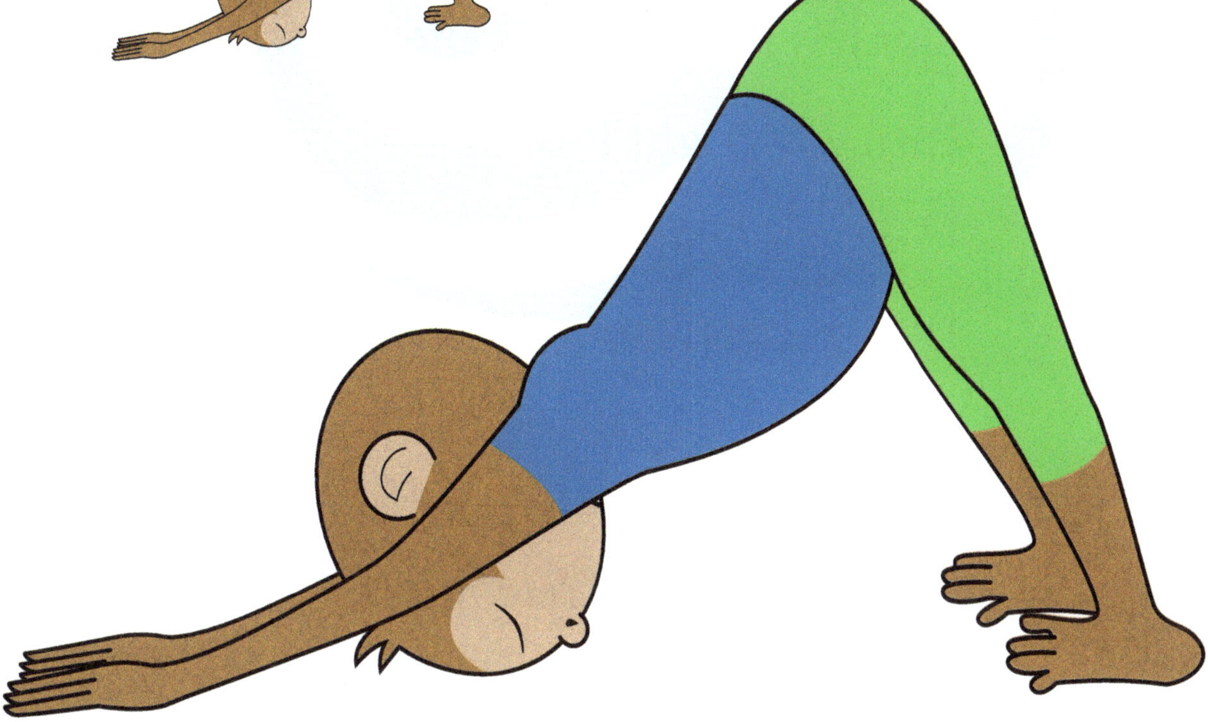

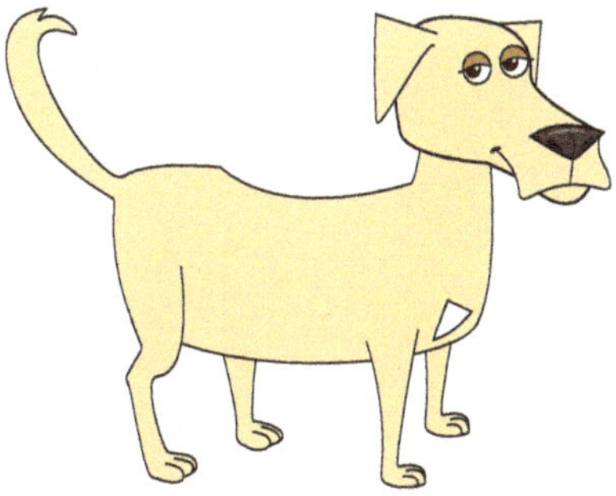

Dogs know this is the best stretch EVER! That's why they named it after us!

DW Dog

Warrior One

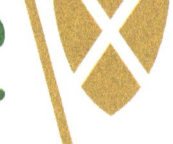

Strong and Balanced

- ☼ Stand with feet together and step your left foot forward about 3 feet.

- ☼ Turn your right foot to a 45 degree angle.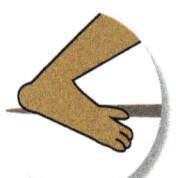

- ☼ Turn at waist and point your hips forward.

- ☼ Sweep your arms up over your head with palms touching.

- ☼ Bend your left knee to a 90 degree angle so it is over your ankle.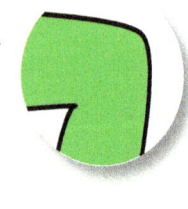

- ☼ Hold for a count of 10! Warriors are strong — you can do it!

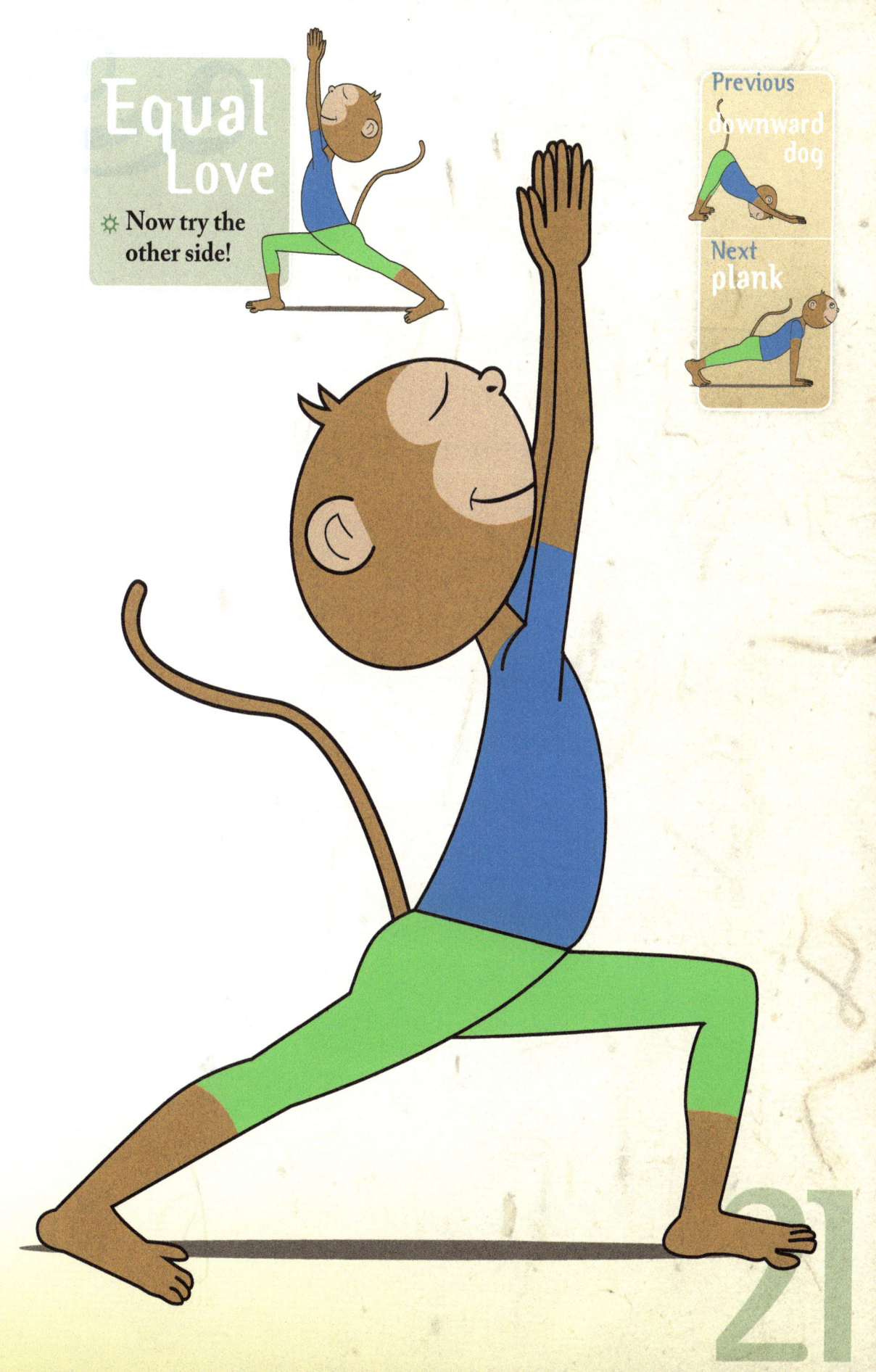

Equal Love

☼ **Now try the other side!**

Previous
downward
dog

Next
plank

21

Plank

Strong and Solid

- ☼ Kneel down on all fours.
- ☼ Hands directly under shoulders.
- ☼ Lift onto toes and straighten legs.
- ☼ Be as straight as a board!
- ☼ Squeeze your belly in and up.
- ☼ Push your heels towards the earth.
- ☼ Lift your head up and smile!

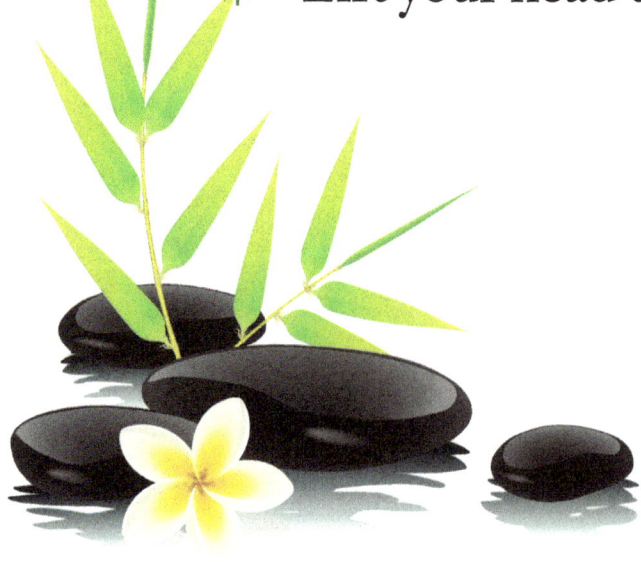

Try-Its

☼ **Drop your knees and do a couple of push-ups, keep elbows close to rib cage.**

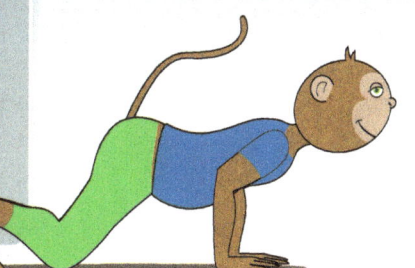

Previous
warrior one

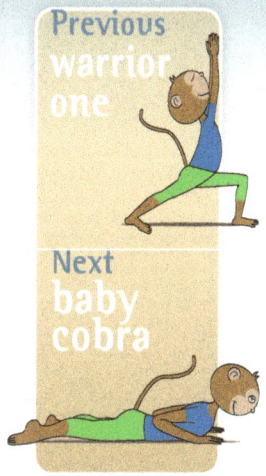

Next
baby cobra

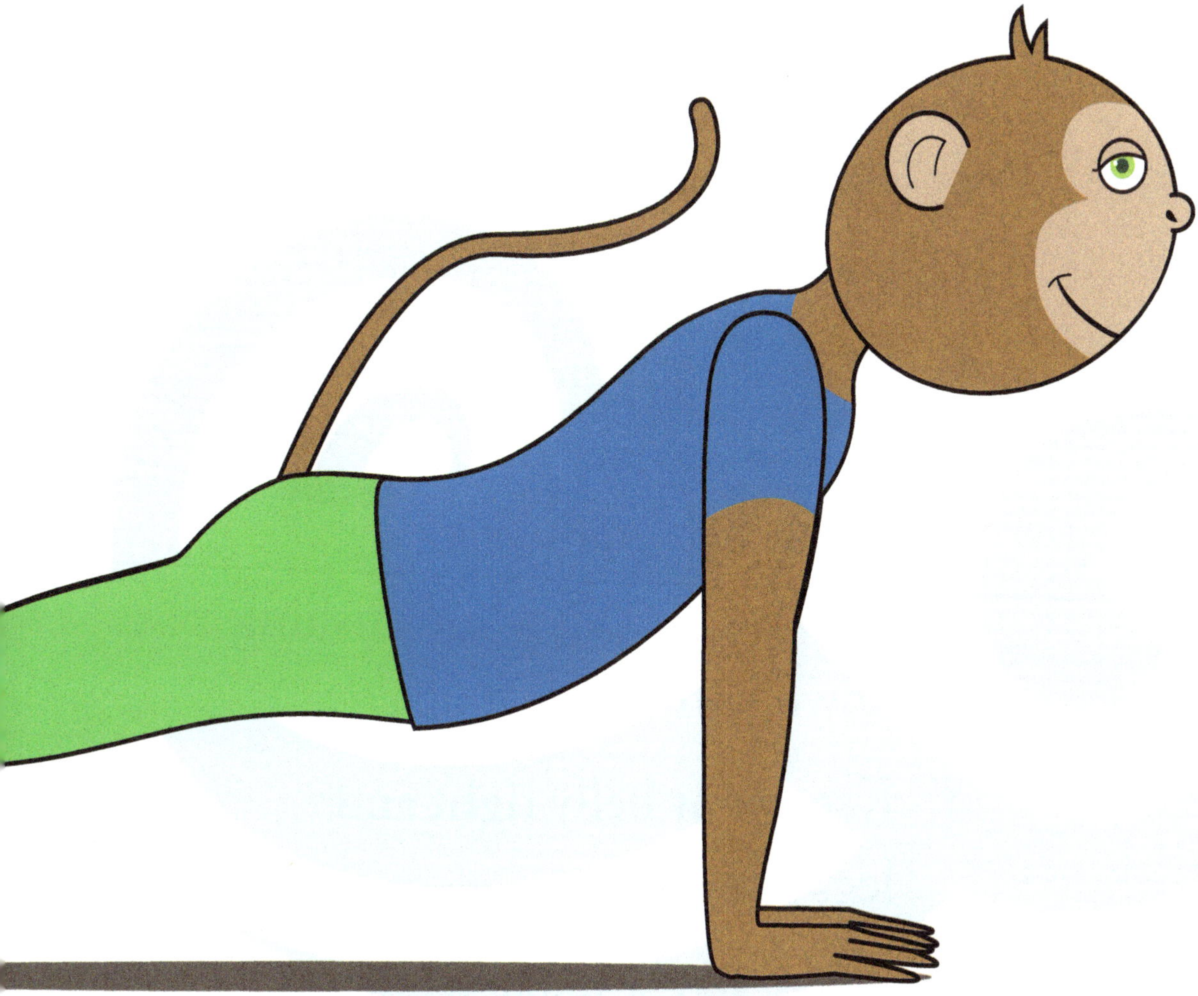

Baby Cobra

Quiet and Intense

- ☼ Begin by lying face down.

- ☼ Press down with the tops of your feet.

- ☼ Place your hands by your shoulders and gently lift your chest forward and up while pushing down with your hands.

- ☼ Keep your belly tight and legs straight.

- ☼ "Hiss" like a snake while you breathe out!

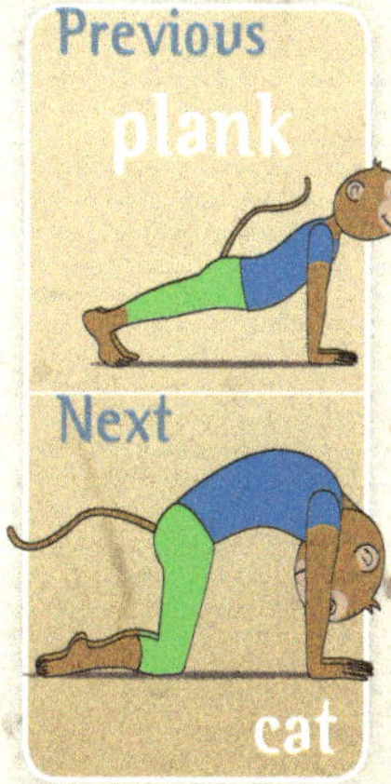

Previous
plank

Next

cat

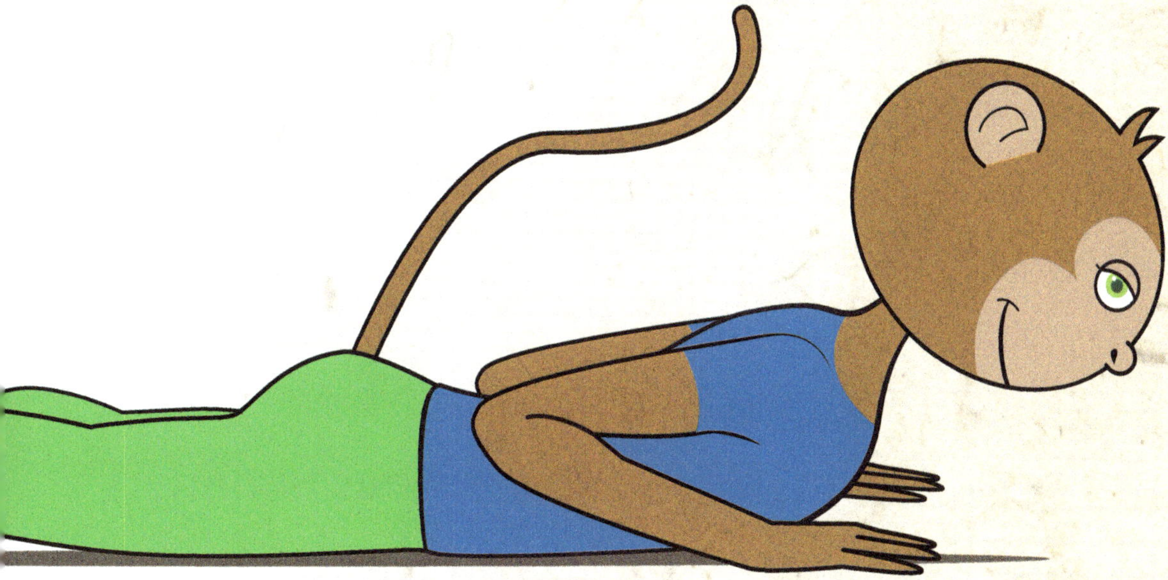

Try-Its

☼ Drop your hands back along your stomach and push your head and shoulders upward. Be the cobra looking for a friend!

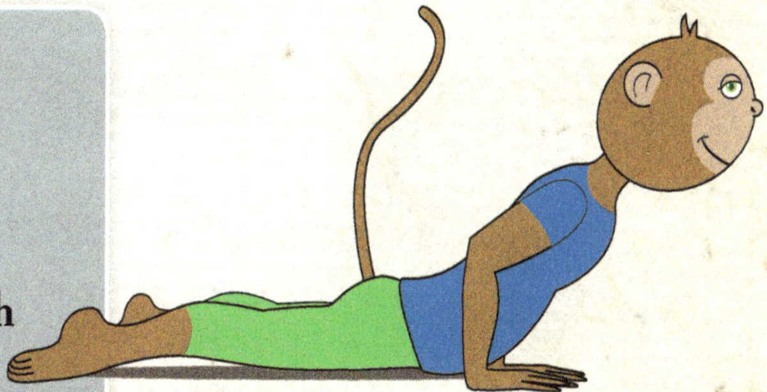

25

Cat

Spirited and Curious

- ☼ Start on hands and knees with your spine straight.

- ☼ Line up your hands under your shoulders and your knees under your hips.

- ☼ On an inhale, squeeze your tummy, round your back as high as you can and drop your head.

- ☼ On your exhale as you release your tummy muscles and come back to a straight spine "meow" like a cat!

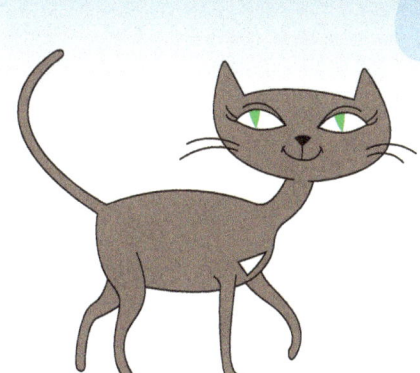

" Arching our back wakes up our sleepy muscles after a cat nap.

Vinka Cat

Previous
baby cobra

Next

cow
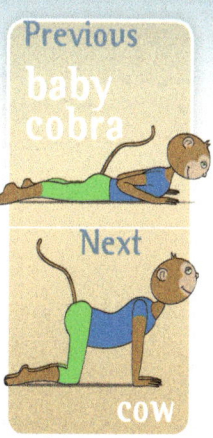

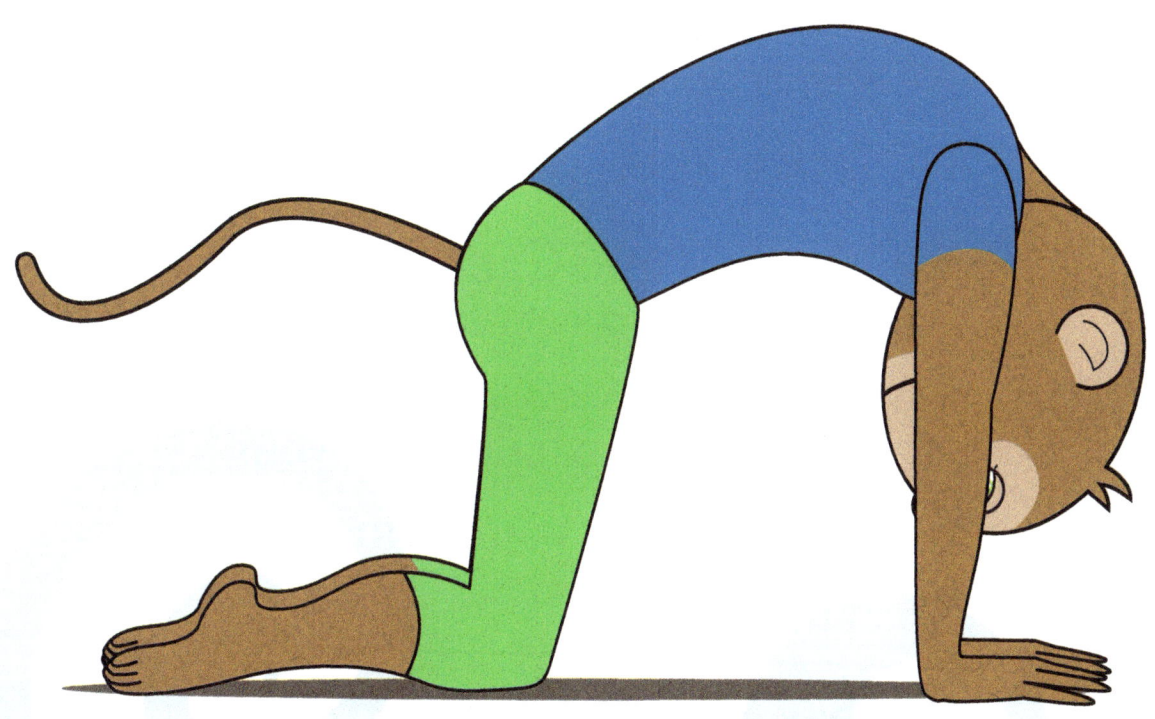

Try-Its

☼ **Do Cat and Cow Pose together.**

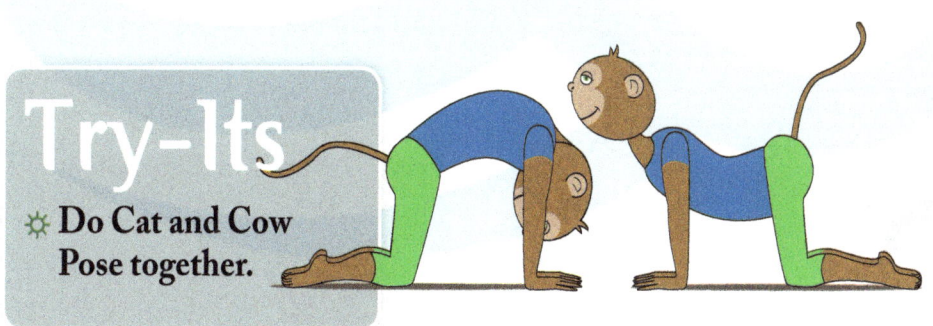

28 Cow

Mellow and Relaxed

☼ Start on all fours, the same as Cat pose.

☼ Arch up into Cat pose on your inhale.

☼ When you exhale, drop your belly and lift your tailbone and head.

☼ Say Moo!

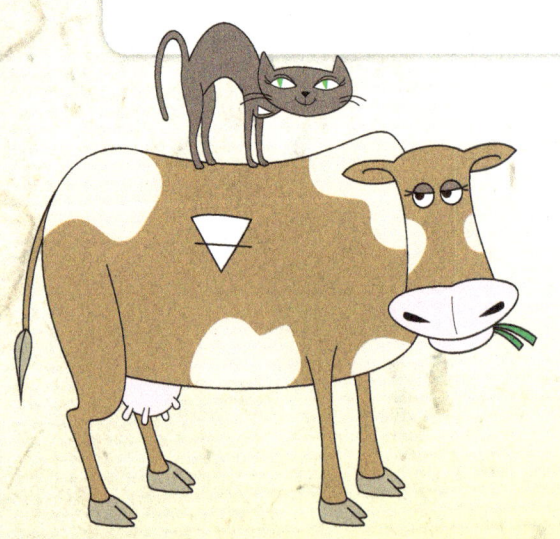

"Cat and I do everything together, she's my best friend.

Belle Cow

Try-Its

☀ **Do Cat and Cow Pose together.**

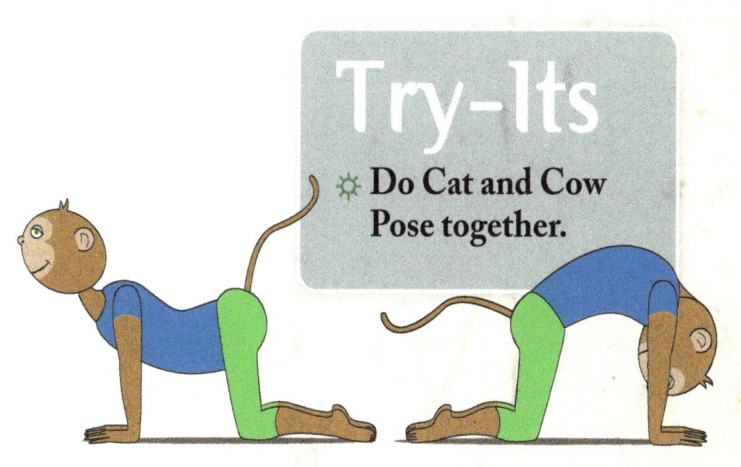

Previous
cat

Next
butterfly

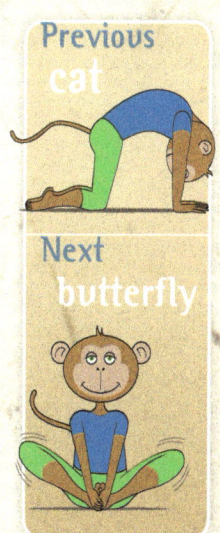

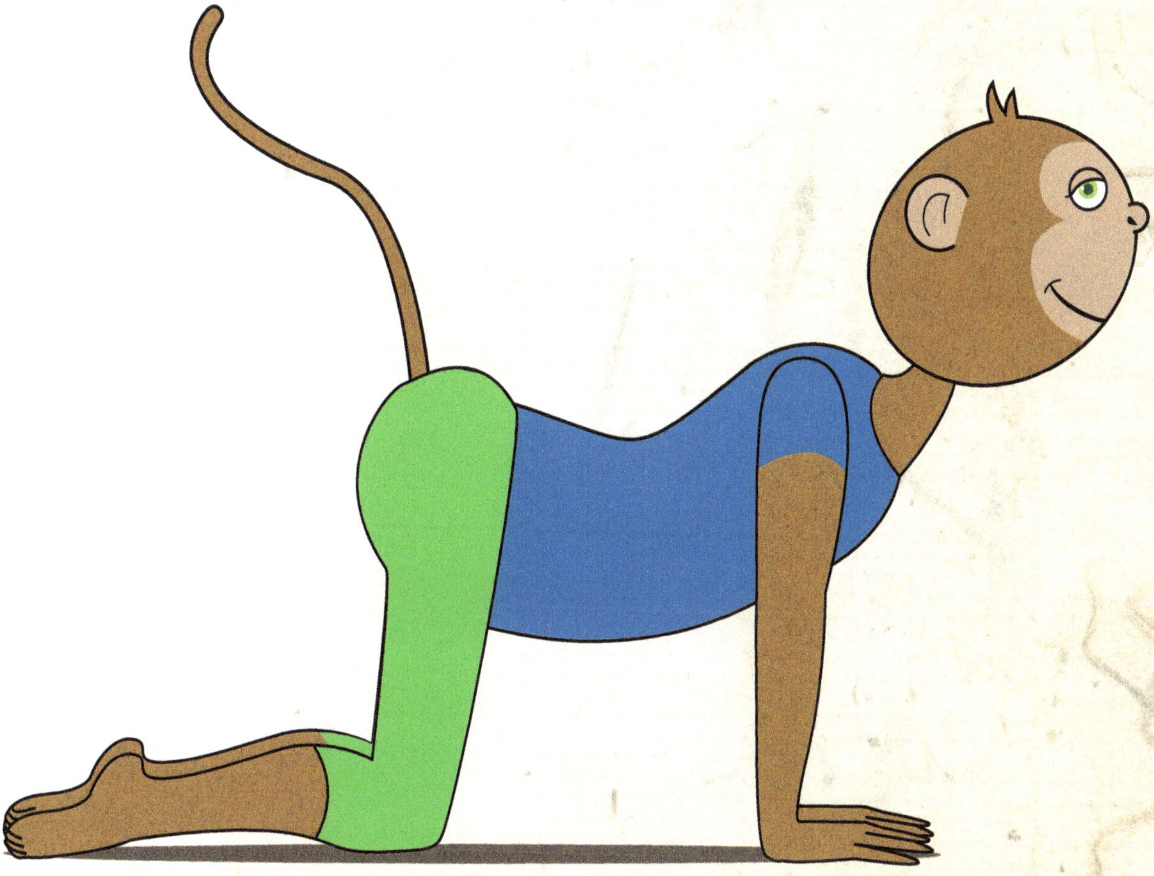

29

Butterfly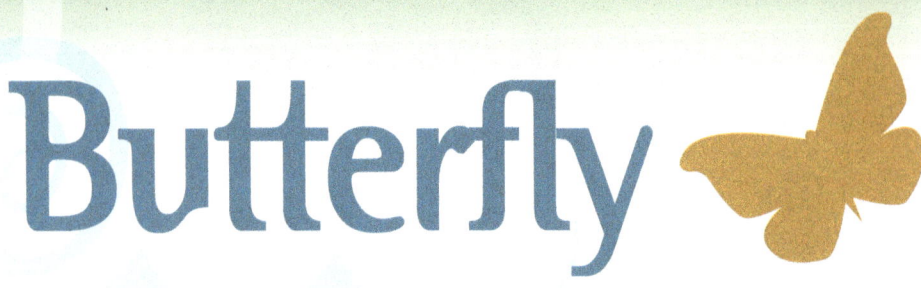

Happy and Free

- ☼ Sit with knees bent and bottoms of feet pressed together.

- ☼ Spine is tall and shoulders are relaxed.

- ☼ Hold your feet and bring them in as close to you as you can.

- ☼ Gently shake legs up and down feeling a stretch in legs and hips.

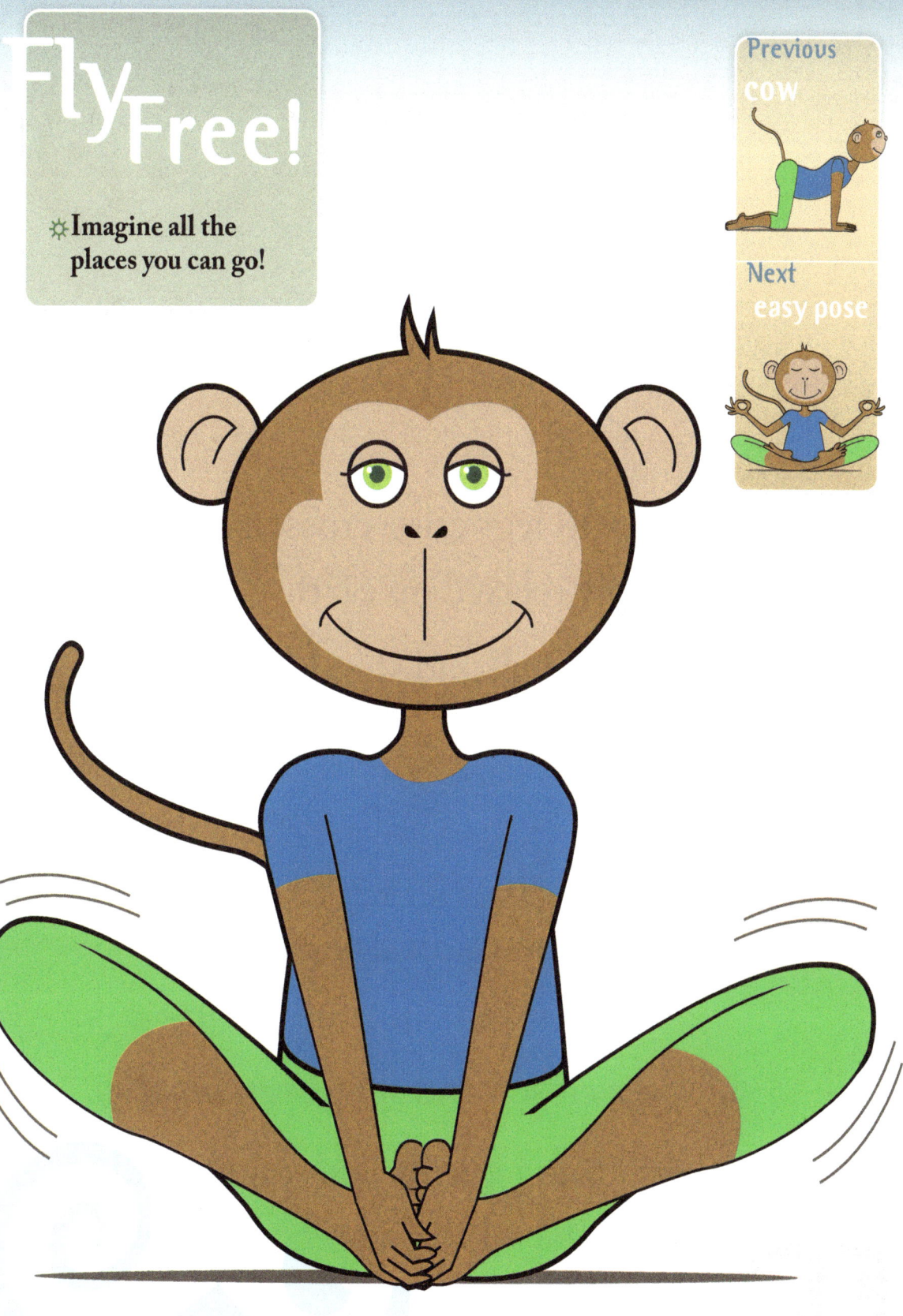

Fly Free!

☼ Imagine all the places you can go!

Previous
cow

Next
easy pose

32 Easy Pose

Grounded and Concentrating

☀ Sit with legs criss-crossed or simply relaxed on earth.

☀ Spine is tall and shoulders are relaxed.

☀ You can put your thumb and pointer finger together to form a circle if you would like, or hands simply resting on your thighs.

☀ Eyes closed and slow even breaths.

☀ Breathing deeply and quietly will quiet the mind and relax the body!

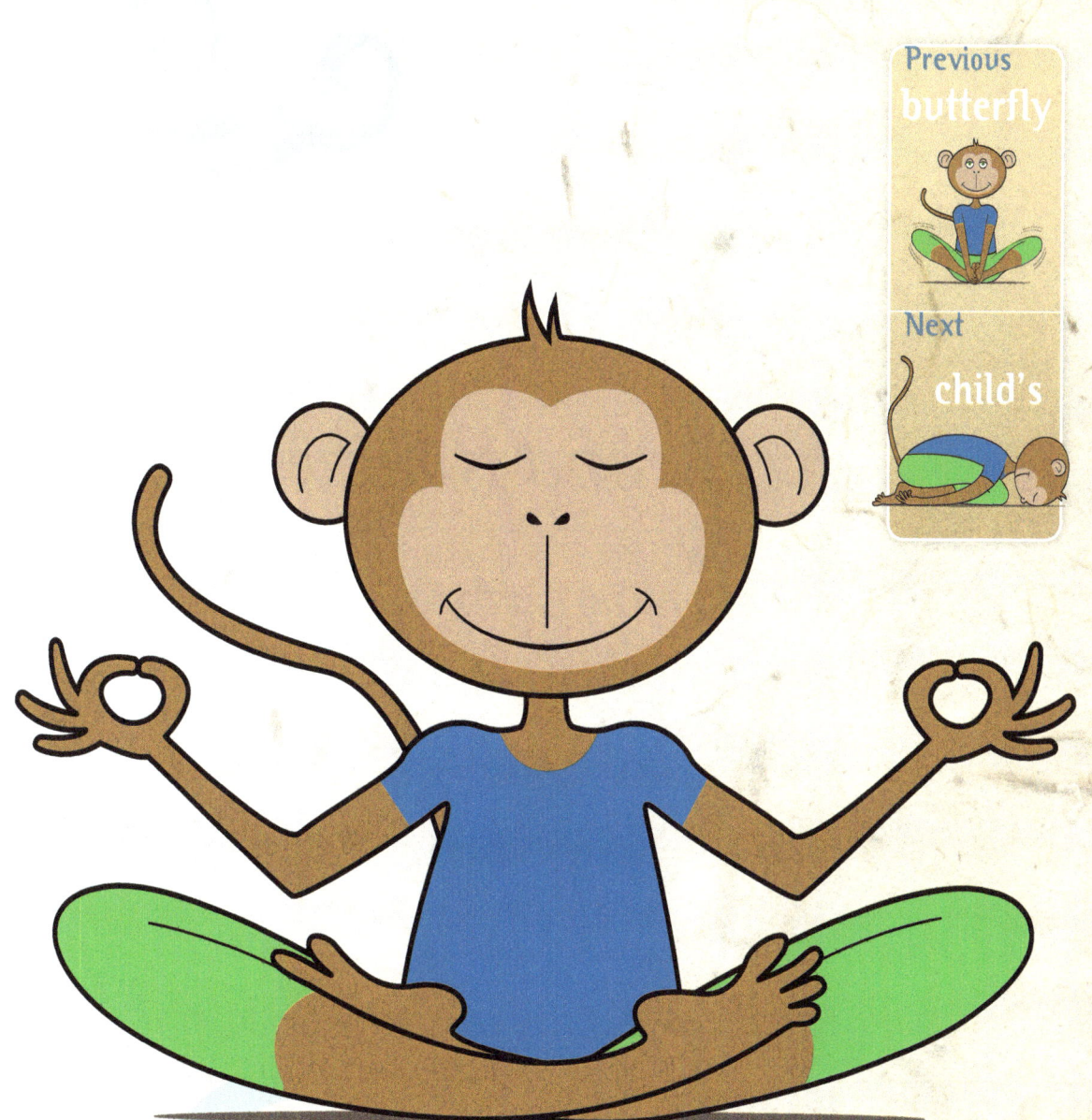

Previous
butterfly

Next
child's

33

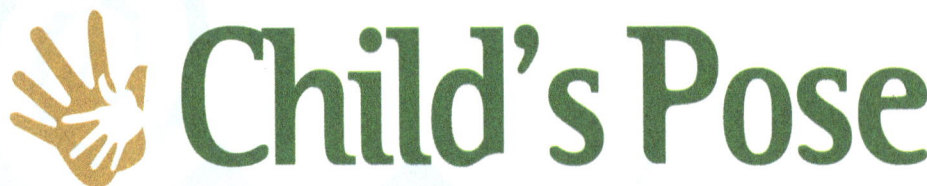

Child's Pose

Relax and Renew

- ☼ Kneel on the earth and bring your bottom towards your heels.

- ☼ With arms at your side, reach your fingertips towards your toes.

- ☼ Gently lower your head to the earth. (A pillow or towel makes it more comfy!)

- ☼ Slowly breathe in and out.

Try Its

☼ This is a relaxation and renewal pose. Try this when you are tired, sad, frustrated or just need a recharge!

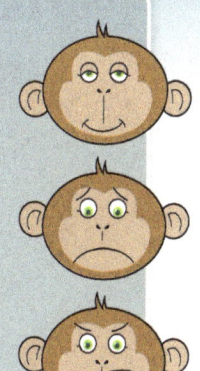

Previous

easy pose

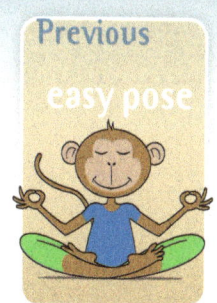

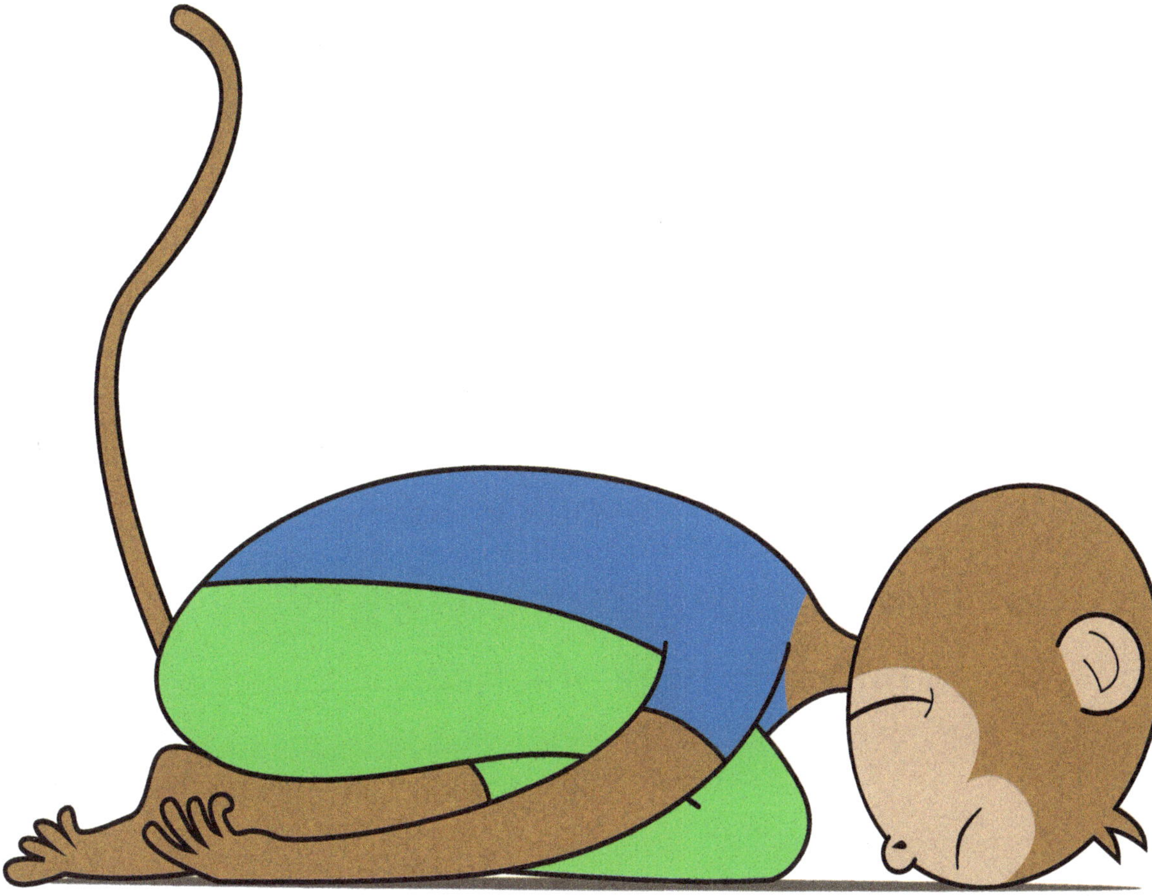

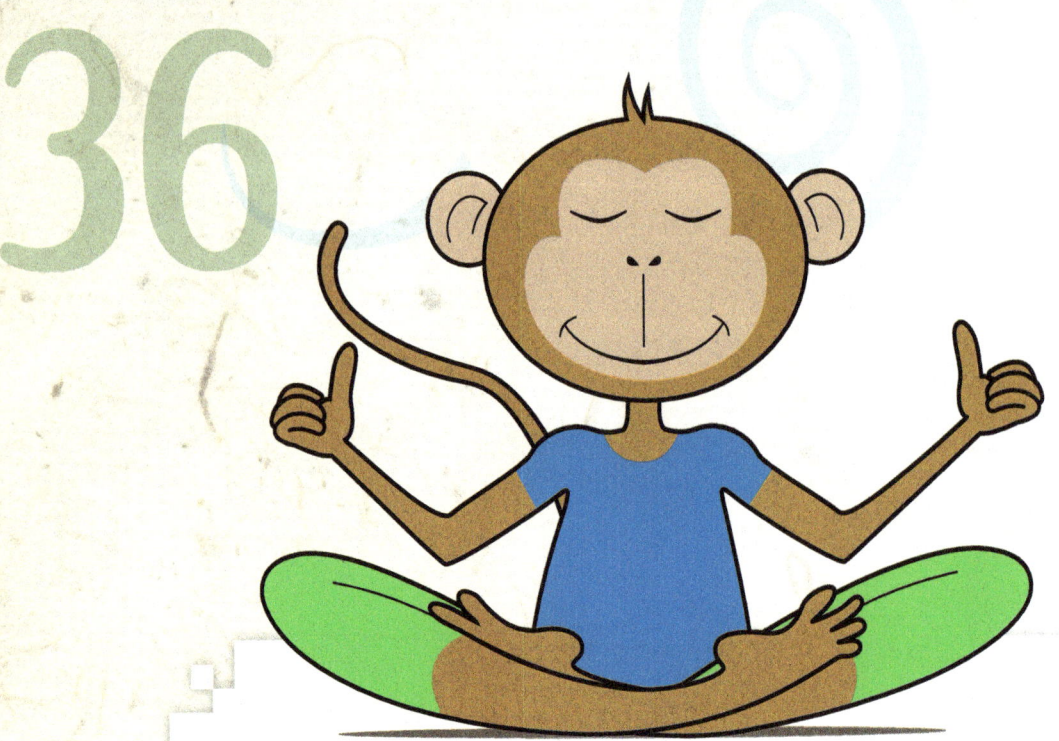

Congratulations! You have learned 12 basic poses. You have started your journey to become a true yogi.

Look for new poses coming out soon to build on your practice.

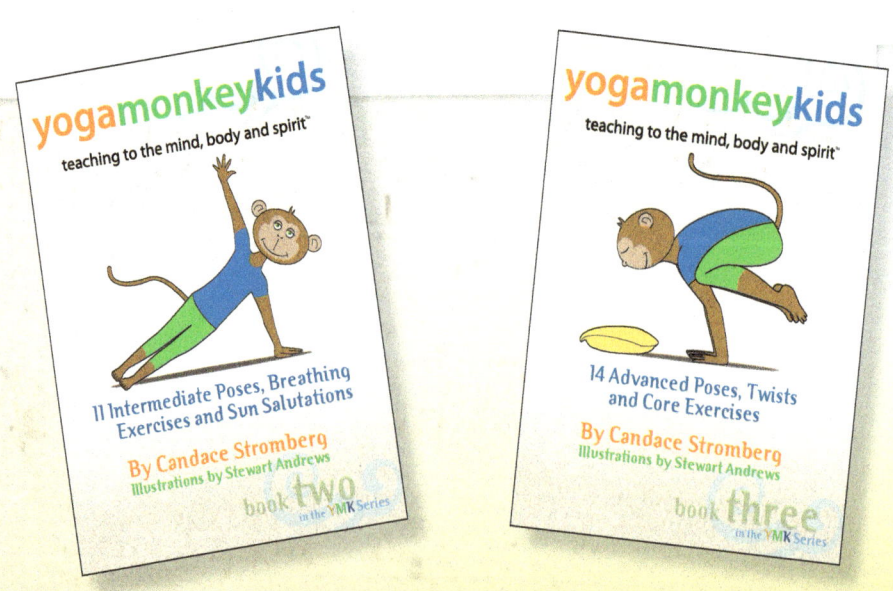

yoga**monkeykids**
teaching to the mind, body and spirit™

11 Intermediate Poses, Breathing Exercises and Sun Salutations

By Candace Stromberg
Illustrations by Stewart Andrews

book **two**
in the YMK Series

yoga**monkeykids**
teaching to the mind, body and spirit™

14 Advanced Poses, Twists and Core Exercises

By Candace Stromberg
Illustrations by Stewart Andrews

book **three**
in the YMK Series

Practice makes progress, not perfect

Remember that yoga is not about being perfect, it's about you being in touch with your body and your thoughts.

Practice the poses often and create your own experience. You can add music and dance. You can practice alone or with family and friends. Bring joy into your practice.

Make your yoga practice as **unique** and **spectacular** as you are!

Get Your Monkey On!

Dedication

For my dad, Donald M. Larrick. I know you are skipping through the galaxy with pride. For all the love, kindness and guidance, I am eternally grateful. I miss you every day.

–C.S.

About the author and creator of Yoga Monkey Kids

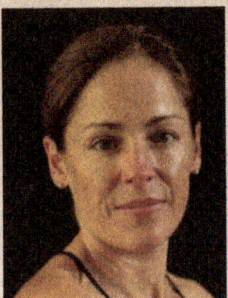

Candace Stromberg has been practicing yoga since 2003 and has been a certified yoga instructor for children since 2010. She has dedicated herself to teaching yoga, nutrition and the integration of mind, body and spirit to kids. That passion for teaching led her to create Yoga Monkey Kids and the family of characters that support her perspective, philosophy and techniques. Yoga Monkey is a labor of love and she feels fortunate to partner with the most wonderful illustrator, designer and dear friend, Stewart Andrews. Her most cherished roles are that of Mom to Daniel and Hannah and wife to Dr. Mark Soberman.

About the Illustrator

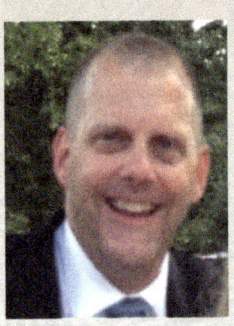

Stewart Andrews is an illustrator and graphic designer who, as a kid, thought nothing of pestering well-known comic strip artists for advice and original drawings. With a BFA in illustration from Virginia Commonwealth University, Stewart is equally fluent creating with a computer or by hand. As a graphic designer with over 30-years of experience, Stewart has an extensive client list spanning several U.S. federal agencies as well as multiple corporations. Stewart's illustrations have garnered multiple awards and have recently been shown at the White House. He lives in McLean, Virginia with his wife, Beth, his two kids, Hanna and Duncan and trusty dachshund, Oakley. See more of Stewart's work at www.noodleboxdesign.com or contact him at stewart@noodleboxdesign.com.

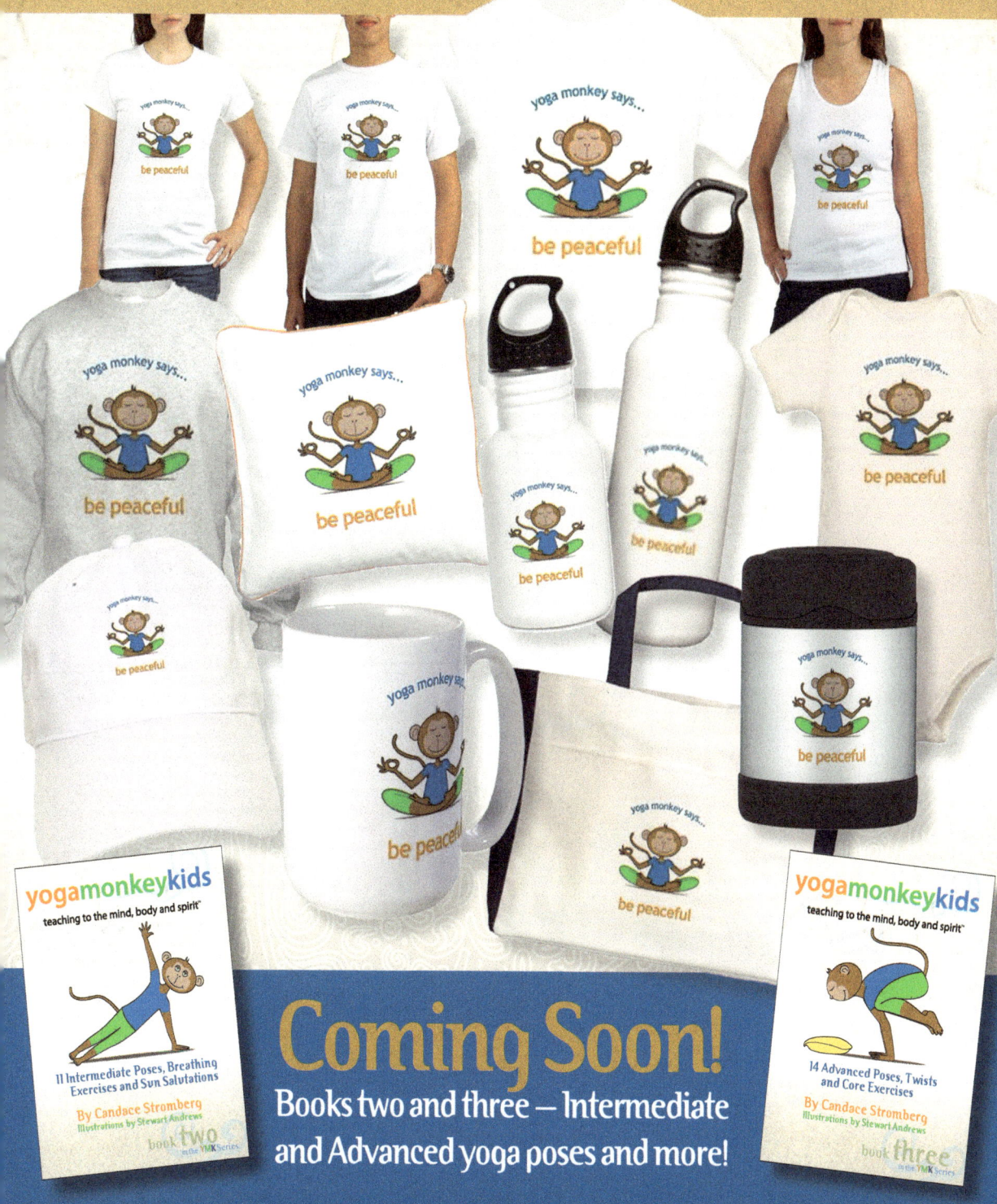

CPSIA information can be obtained
at www.ICGtesting.com
Printed in the USA
BVOW10s0823171116
468164BV00011B/18/P

9 781683 487524